Regaining Bladder Control

*For incontinence on exertion
or following pelvic surgery*

by Eileen Montgomery
M.C.S.P.

Second Edition

Clinical Press

© Copyright Clinical Press

All Rights Reserved. No part of this publication may be reproduced, stored in a retrieval system, or transmitted in any form or by any means, electronic, mechanical, photocopying, recording or otherwise, without the prior permission of the copyright owner.

ISBN 1 85457 003X

First published 1974
Revised reprint 1983
Reprinted 1985
Second edition 1989

Published by Clinical Press Ltd.,
Registered address: 'The Coach House',
26 Oakfield Road, Clifton, Bristol,
BS8 2AT, England

Printed in Great Britain by Manor Printing Services (Wotton) Ltd.,
Kingswood, Wotton-under-Edge, Glos

FOREWORD

Far too many people unfortunately suffer from the occasional unintentional leakage of urine. Of the various types of urinary loss, stress incontinence is one of the commonest, often starting quite unexpectedly or perhaps following surgery or childbirth; the leak occurs on exertion when playing games, running, jumping, or merely on coughing, laughing or sneezing. Whatever the circumstances, the onset of this condition can be a devastating experience for the individual irrespective of the amount of leakage, undermining self-confidence and causing a depressing prospect for the future. All too often the immediate reaction is a completely negative one, with avoidance of any activity that might precipitate further leakage and a reluctance to seek advice. Exercise is curtailed, fluids are restricted and a pad is worn for protection. Thus the vicious circle is established, body weight increases and the pelvic muscles are allowed to become yet weaker.

Eileen Montgomery provides an alternative approach, a positive attitude to this problem, focusing directly on the weakness of the pelvic muscles. Her enthusiasm and commitment for teaching somehow stimulates her patients to use muscles that they had never realised even existed. Many people do want to help themselves and this book provides clear instructions for them to follow. First they must understand that anatomy of the pelvic floor muscles, then learn how to use them and finally possess the self-discipline to perform the exercises regularly every day. So many patients have been cured by this simple course of treatment, hence avoiding surgery that yet a further edition of her book has been requested and produced. My one plea is that those who suffer from this problem study her method at the time of its onset rather than 10 years later.

Roger Feneley, Consultant Urologist,
Southmead Hospital, Bristol

MOST PEOPLE, except in infancy and perhaps in senility, control their bladders satisfactorily without undue worry. The outflow is suppressed until it can occur at an appropriate time and place.

This little book is not intended for them—unless a relation, or somebody in whom they are interested, has a tendency to leak. It has been written to help adults who are able to control the outflow most of the time, but have lost the ability to do so on effort, such as when they cough, sneeze, lift heavy weights or jump. These people have a problem which, more often than not, they themselves can overcome. This book will tell them how to do it and also help others to hasten the return to normal function following either pelvic surgery or medical treatment for specific urinary disorders. Some people have a too-frequently desire to pass water (which may be due to inflammation of the bladder) and some have sudden uncontrollably strong urges to do so owing to overactivity of the bladder's expulsive muscle. With cause traced and proper medical treatment, these symptoms can be cured or controlled—so they should consult their doctor without delay. Re-education along the following lines may then be all-important.

We must eliminate at the very beginning those people whose difficulties are of a type unlikely to be helped by the techniques about to be described. They are incontinent men and women, in whom the imperfection is in the nervous system. The brain may have been damaged or the nerve pathways blocked, so that impulses cannot get through to the bladder. There may be no sensory alarm signal as the bladder fills with urine. These people are deprived of the power of control while the paralysis exists. Half the problem is knowing who to ask for advice to make their condition as comfortable and acceptable as possible. In many cases, after observation and training with whoever is responsible for their care, they are able to regulate voiding so that it occurs *before* the bladder is full to overflowing—and so remain dry. (See *Appendix.*)

Exertion (or Stress) Incontinence

This is the name given to the type which can be cured. It is commoner than one might think, because sufferers do not, as a rule, talk about it, except to their family and closest friends. It is an embarrassment which presents itself damply and uncomfortably, but only on exertion: the stress is mechanical, not emotional.

It often constrains the personality. The pleasantest of people tend to become less sociable and more inhibited in their manner if they suffer from this complaint. In company their enjoyment can be ruined!

Many sufferers have already sought medical assistance for their persistent dampness, only to be told 'You'll have to learn to live with it!' This remark could be taken to mean either 'You'll have to learn to put up with it', or 'There is nothing more that can be done about it'. Whichever way it is taken, this conclusion is very depressing, but it is just not true.

A New Approach to Cure

Recently, we have developed an approach which is dependent, not on the skills of others, but on one's own tenacity—given the know-how. It is a form of self-discipline by which, with patience and the will to follow through a course of exercises, perfect control of the bladder can be regained.

To solve a problem, one must understand it; so first of all, we must discuss this one in more detail.

The Cause of the Trouble

Weakness of the supportive muscles underneath the bladder is the cause of the trouble. It is a law of nature that the efficient functioning of every part of a living body is maintained or improved through constant use. In this way, all the species on earth have evolved and adapted to their own special pattern of existence and survival. Conversely, if any anatomical feature is *not used,* it will become enfeebled and eventually waste away. People who do not exercise their faculties, lose them.

Nowadays, athletes who injure or strain a muscle know full well that they may never regain their peak of performance if they allow the injured part to be immobilized for long. They are encouraged by their trainers to get back into action as soon as possible—before muscle atrophy sets in.

After an illness, when there has been a period of enforced and necessary rest, patients should begin to activate their muscles as soon as possible—moderately at first—to restore their tone before they get back to the old routine.

On returning to consciousness after an operation, patients are persuaded to try—and keep on trying—to move gently, even if it does hurt! If they fail to do so, the muscles become less effective within a short time.

This fact of life has not always been appreciated. Not so very long ago, it was regarded as being of the utmost importance for people to remain motionless during the period of healing.

Women who are now unable to prevent the escape of urine under increased stress, may have had a period of complete inactivity within the pelvis, at some time in their lives—perhaps following childbirth or pelvic surgery. Soft tissues might have been overstretched or incised and stitched, resulting in some reluctance to move, afterwards. The whole area could have remained clogged, swollen and inert for days. In consequence, the pelvic muscles may have become flabby and unable to contract sufficiently to compress the outlet tube from the bladder (urethra), as once they did.

Men may have had a similar period of rest following surgery to the prostate gland or bladder. The condition is sometimes brought on by faulty postural habits which are often associated with being overweight.

All movements are produced by muscles. They do it (when ordered to by the brain via the nervous system) by contracting their elastic fibres and drawing closer the structures to which they are attached. When released, they are softer and more yielding. But overstretched muscles react like boiled elastic—and may be just as useless!

Yet, even though unpleasant symptoms have been endured for years, it is possible for those flagging muscles to be coaxed into becoming effective stop taps again. The exercises which are described later have helped many women to do this. They should also be done to hasten a return to full function, following pelvic surgery in both men and women.

Our control of the skeletal muscles—which are concerned with everything we *do*—is conscious (voluntary), while that of the muscles which regulate our essential functions, e.g. breathing, circulation of blood, digestion, fluid balance, elimination of waste

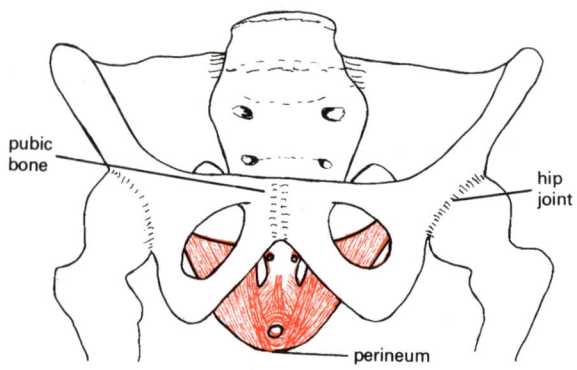

Fig. 1. The pelvis viewed from the front, showing the pelvic floor muscles slung from it like a hammock.

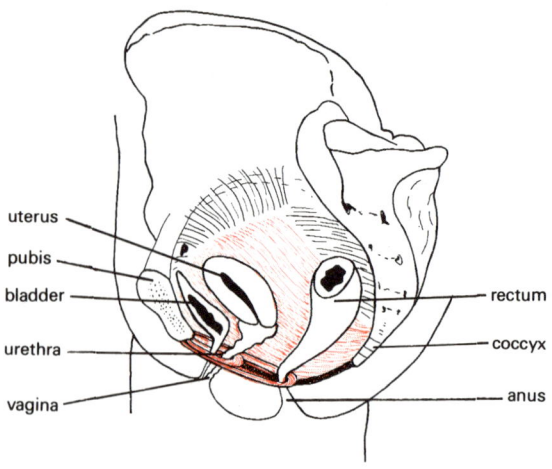

Fig. 2. The right part of the female pelvic cavity, showing in red the main muscle sheet of the pelvic floor and the 'straps' one of which loops around the anus, and the other around the vagina and urethra.

products etc. is unconscious (involuntary). Muscles of *both* types play their part in the control of our pelvic organs.

The Structures of the Pelvic Area

The pelvis is the girdle of bone which forms the framework of the lower part of the trunk. In shape, it is like a basin with a hole in its base. Stretched across the hole cradling the organs within the basin are the muscles of the pelvic floor (*Fig.* 1).

The bladder is situated inside the pelvic basin, towards the front; the rectum (where waste food products collect) lies at the back; while in women, the uterus (womb) rests between the two, in the middle (*Fig.* 2).

The Pelvic Floor Muscles

The pelvic floor muscles form a hammock composed of interweaving contractile fibres, which is attached at the back to the coccyx (the 'tail-bones' at the base of the spine) and in the front to the pubis (which can be felt below the 'tummy' wall).

Imagine a garden hammock, slung between two trees. One could pull it up or let it down from either end. In the same way, our pelvic 'hammock' can be drawn up at will, when the muscle fibres are contracted, or let down when they are relaxed—from either attachment or both at the same time—and the angle at which it is slung can be altered accordingly.

The genital and outlet tubes pass through the 'hammock' and at these places, the fibres divide to by-pass them. These gaps are the areas of maximal strain, and since women have three openings and men only two it will be obvious why the female is more vulnerable than the male!

R. H. Paramore and Sir Arthur Keith described in their Hunterian Lectures how the pelvic floor muscles have played a most interesting part in human evolution. At a very primitive stage, they merely moved the tail; but as tails were used less and less, they degenerated. The muscles then began to change and undertook the more specialized duty of regulating the pressure within the abdomen, which varies on forced respiration and on straining to excrete from the pelvis.

Later still, when our forefathers adopted the upright posture for locomotion, work and play, the muscles were entrusted with counteracting the pull of gravity and supporting the internal organs.

Nowadays, many people are still capable of depressing and (to a slight degree) wagging what is left of their tails (the coccyx). Performing tail movements helps to strengthen the pelvic floor for its more important supportive role. It is significant to note that monkeys—also upright creatures spending a great deal of their time on two legs—who have retained their long tails and use them frequently, do not seem to suffer from stress incontinence!

The pelvic floors of four-footed animals are not called upon to take the same amount of strain. They stand and run about with their bodies in a prone position, and the weight of their internal organs is borne by a bony shelf of pubis and their abdominal walls.

Think of the abdomen as a cylinder containing those organs; the pelvic floor as its base and the dome-shaped diaphragm its top, which works like a plumber's plunger when respiratory, expulsive and other physical efforts are made. As the diaphragm moves down, the pressure in the abdomen goes up, making an impact on the pelvic floor and organs.

However, nature has done her best to help mankind to adapt to excessive strain. Dissections by J. O. N. Lawson, F.R.C.S. show that we have developed two strap-like slings of muscle to give greater security. From the pubis on the left and right of midline, one loops around the urethra and vagina, the other around the junction of the lower bowel with the anus. When they contract, they squeeze those tubes and pull them up and forward. When the stress (pressure) is raised—on laughing, sneezing, coughing, lifting, hitting a ball or whatever—they should contract spontaneously, one guarding against an escape of urine by compressing the urethra and the other guarding against leakage of gas or excrement from the anus. (See *Fig. 2.*)

The Bladder

The bladder is a reservoir for collecting urine. It has an internal sphincter (a ring-shaped muscle which acts like a mechanical valve) around its neck, where it joins the urethra. This mechanism, which is *not* controlled by the will, usually works efficiently while the pressure within the bladder is low, particularly when one is lying down. But as it fills up and the pressure is raised, it needs reinforcement. The pelvic floor muscles are then called upon to go into action, voluntarily.

So what needs to be done if your Reservoir Leaks on Exertion?

1. The pelvic floor muscles—the secondary line of defence—need retraining and strengthening, so that they become competent at stopping the escape of urine.

2. There may be parts of your body 'engine' which are functioning imperfectly and thereby contributing to the weakness in your pelvic suspension. If so, your attention must be directed towards improving their condition, too.

Would you expect a motor, with coked-up cylinders or an inefficient exhaust system, to get a car—fully loaded—to your destination without a hitch? Of course not! You would get it serviced by an expert before driving it on a long journey.

Check for any Predisposing Mechanical Faults

1. Get coughs cured as quickly as possible. Each one is like a bounce on the pelvic floor.

2. Steer clear of constipation. Straining down on an already-weakened pelvic hammock may tax its strength beyond the limit it is able to withstand.

3. Avoid overloading the 'springs' by carrying excessive weight, or this may have a similar effect.

Should you need advice on how to overcome any of these three contributive conditions, you will find it towards the end of the book. Let us deal with the main problem first.

To Regain Command over the Bladder under Stress

The aims are:

1. To develop awareness of body and posture. For this, one must *concentrate* while performing the prescribed movements, so that feelings are registered in the mind.

2. To increase the strength and reactions of all the weak muscles; especially those inner ones which lift the pelvic floor and close the urethra. Also the muscles which stabilize the pelvis as it rocks on the hip joints.

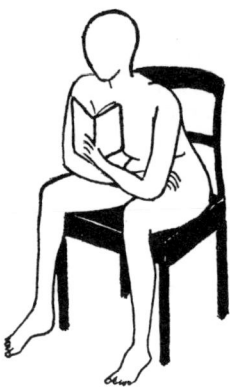

Fig. 3. Basic position for pelvic floor exercises. Let both forearms rest on thighs when book is not needed.

When the exercises are done as a routine, the numerous involuntary muscles in and around the pelvic organs are influenced to perform better, as cardiac muscles are with graded activity in a scheme of rehabilitation after heart failure. The above effects are achieved with extra benefits: the joints of the pelvis, hips and lower spine become more supple, circulation is improved and stagnant tissues are revived with oxygenated blood.

All these factors combine to bring about a more healthy and responsive state. Nerves and muscles, which previously interacted rather sluggishly, begin to react to each other more briskly.

Drinking eight to ten cups of liquid daily is recommended. If the fluid intake is reduced in the mistaken belief that it will reduce the leakage, the urine becomes too strong, irritating the bladder.

The Basic Exercises for the Pelvic Floor Muscles

To be Repeated FREQUENTLY during the Day

Sit well back on a chair, thighs and feet supported, knees comfortably apart. Lean forward, forearms on thighs, book in hand (*Fig.* 3). Concentrate.

Begin by lifting the pelvic 'hammock' from its back attachments:

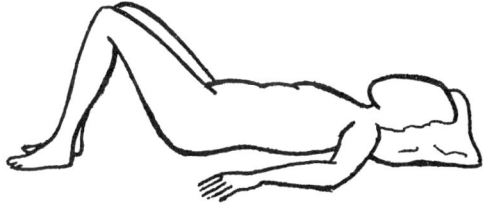

Fig. 4. Lying position for pelvic floor exercises.

MOVEMENT 1

From the 'tail' bones, slowly pull up the central, lowest point of the muscle (the perineum—the part between the back and front passages). Register the feeling of the underbody being drawn towards the base of the spine inside the pelvis. Feel the tension, firming and tightening, between the perineum and the 'tail', as the muscle contracts to lift upwards and backwards.

Relax. Feel the muscles softening and slackening with the descent.

NB You should not have been contracting the buttocks.

Draw up the 'hammock' towards your 'tail' a second time, and make sure that tension and slight uplift are felt inside only, towards the back of the pelvis.

Now lift the pelvic floor up from its front attachments, contracting those muscular 'straps' which loop around the outlet tubes:

MOVEMENT 2

Place finger tips on the top of the pubic hair line. Pull the perineum up towards the pubis behind your fingers.

NB Do not contract the muscles on the inside of the thigh.

Feel the central and forward part of the underbody being caught up and compressed towards the front of the pelvis, inside. Register in your mind the sensation of tension produced behind the pubis.

Go on . . . just a bit more . . . to the limit of movement.

Let go. Notice how soft and slack it feels by contrast, when completely relaxed.

Repeat it, slowly, without the finger touch this time. Do not involve the 'tummy' muscles or press the thighs together. At this

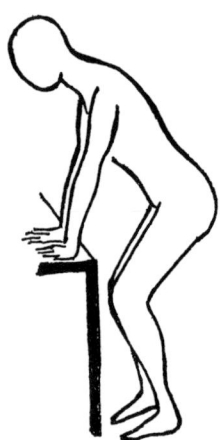

Fig. 5. Standing position for pelvic floor exercise.

stage of your muscular re-education, contractions of muscles outside the pelvis may obscure your perception of genuine pelvic floor activity. Register that feeling of tension in the muscle fibres towards the *front* of the pelvic floor with the compression of the urinary outlet. *This is the all-important action which closes the stop-tap.*

Relax again. Feel the muscles slacken.

Yet, it does take concentration, but it will get easier with practice! Make sure that you give your perceptive senses time to get the message and record the different feelings in the brain.

Weak pelvic floor muscles tire fairly quickly; so at first it will be enough to perform each movement five times at one go—but increase gradually to ten and try to practice them at least every hour that you are awake.

When you have mastered the actions in sitting forward, do them on some occasions in alternative positions—but still with the hips bent. This is important because it is easier to localize the muscular activity and to appreciate exactly what is happening *inside* the pelvis, when in this position.

Do them:

1. In bed, lying on back or side, with knees crooked up (*Fig.* 4).

2. Kneeling on all fours (*see Fig.* 6).

3. Standing, leaning forwards from the hips with hands flat on the table—a sort of 'giraffe' position (*Fig.* 5).

After One Week

Combine movements 1 and 2—Lying, sitting or standing. Pull the perineum up towards the 'tail' then, holding it tightly, pull forward and up towards the pubis and squeeze as hard as possible.

Imagine a string running down inside you from the navel, through your abdomen and pelvis, to the perineum. Pretend to pull up the string inside towards the navel.

Do it slowly . . . up . . . up to the limit (taking about five seconds to do it).

Relax.

When pulling up, you should not feel any tension in the buttocks or the 'tummy' muscles. If you do, you are cheating!

The point of the exercise is to re-train yourself to *use* the pelvic floor muscles properly. Form the habit of contracting them at certain times and with regular happenings: standing up from a lying, reclining or sitting position, cleaning teeth, taking a bath, talking on the telephone, washing the dishes, cooking, lifting, or just waiting at the supermarket check-out—for anything or anybody. Give yourself cues.

Eventually, if you keep up this routine activity, you will be able to do it without that glassy-eyed look of concentration and then— since nobody will know what you are doing—you should find yourself able to pull up inside while conversing, in any position, whenever it comes to mind.

'Tappers Drill'

This exercise should be performed when intentionally emptying the bladder:

Start the urine flow . . . and try to stop in midstream by pulling the pelvic floor muscles upwards and forwards to squeeze the urethra.

Start the stream again . . . and when voiding is completed, pull up strongly and hold for five seconds.

At first, you may find it impossible to stop completely when the bladder needs emptying rather urgently; but go on trying. It will get easier as the pelvic muscles strengthen.

Anticipation and the Counter-brace

This is of the utmost importance. Train yourself to brace up before taking strain. If you are about to lift, push, cough, laugh, blow, sneeze or do any action which causes a downward thrust, be on your guard!

Prepare yourself to take the increased stress by contracting your pelvic floor, gripping the urethra and holding it tightly until the exertion is over.

Now that the action of the pelvic floor muscles is understood better, it must be obvious that if the pressure from within the abdomen and the bladder is increased suddenly without any increase in the resistance—a leakage is almost inevitable!

So you simply must get into the habit of adopting a posture of defence when those muscles are threatened from within.

Exercises for the Pelvic Floor; plus the Stabilizing Postural Muscles on the Outer Sides of the Pelvis

These movements should be performed once a day.

Kneeling

Kneeling on hands and knees. Imagine that you are a dog, with a long tail stretched out behind you (*Fig.* 6).

1. Tuck that tail down and underneath you, slowly, until it is pointing towards your chin.

Feel the buttock muscles contracting to pull the pelvis down at the back, while the abdominal muscles are contracting to draw the pubis up closer to the ribs in front (back rounded) (*Fig.* 7).

Relax and return to the starting position—tail stretched out behind. Repeat five times and then rest.

2. Raise the tail slowly until it is pointing up to the ceiling (back hollowed at the waist) (*Fig.* 8).

Relax and return to the starting position.

Repeat five times and rest with head down on the forearms for a few moments.

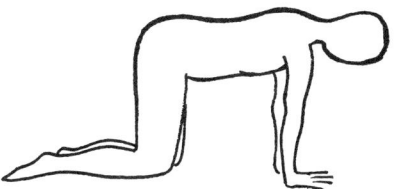

Fig. 6. The starting position on all fours.

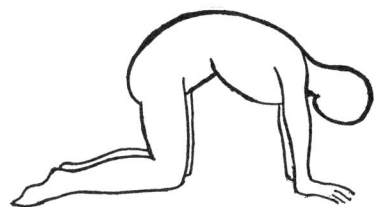

Fig. 7. Depressing the tail.

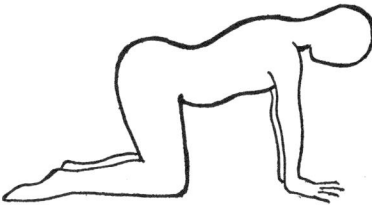

Fig. 8. Raising the tail.

Up on hands and knees again, or if this starting position puts a strain on your wrists, do the movements instead kneeling, but resting your forearms on a low stool, sofa, divan or chair, with head on hands and back horizontal.

If you should be unable to kneel, then stand to do them, with hips and knees slightly bent, and lean over, as in *Fig.* 6 but with the forearms instead of palms resting on a table.

3. Wag the tail to the left—slowly—to the limit of movement (*Fig.* 9).

Then to the right.

Repeat smoothly five times, wagging as far as possible each way.

Relax and rest for a few moments.

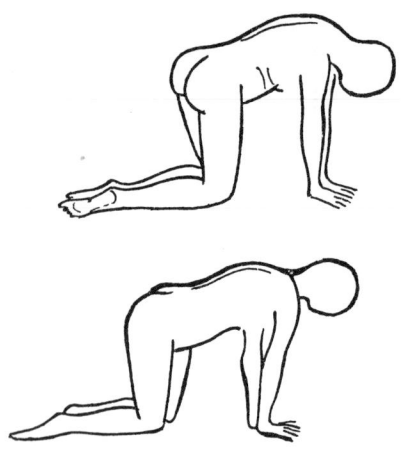

Fig. 9. Wagging the tail.

4. Circle the tail. Up . . . left . . . down . . . right . . . up . . . and repeat three times. Then do it in the other direction, up . . . right . . . down . . . left . . . up . . . and repeat three times. Rest.

Upright

CHECK AND READJUST YOUR POSTURE WHEN STANDING

Lean against a wall with heels six inches (15 cm.) away from it. Iron out the hollow of your back by pressing your waist backwards. Feel all your spinal bones touching the wall from tail to shoulders (*Fig.* 10).

Think about the position of your spine and hips. Then relax.

Remember that when muscles are subjected to cumulative strain their natural elasticity and sensitivity are reduced to a great extent. Your day-to-day working habits can affect your disability.

One should not stand with a forward-tilted pelvis, a hollow back and a bulging tummy or the 'hammock' suspended inside the pelvis is also tilted forward. There is then a tendency for the bladder neck to fall on (and possibly through) the gap where there is no supportive muscle tissue near the front of the pelvic floor (*See Fig.* 1).

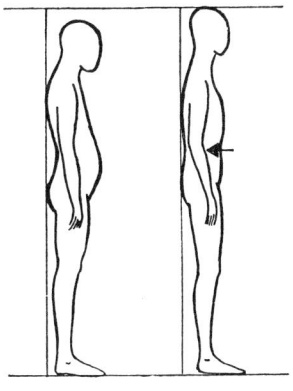

Fig. 10.

STAND AWAY FROM THE WALL AND READJUST AGAIN

Feet parallel. Body weight spread evenly between the heels and the balls of the feet. Bend the knees slightly to reduce excessive tension in the legs. Rock your pubis up and forwards from the hip joints. Hold your waist back, your tummy in and your seat down. Straighten your knees *gently* and relax, allowing the pelvis to balance itself in a position of stability and comfort (tail in mid-range).

Make sure that your pelvis is balanced—like a boat on a calm sea—then try to lift your body up out of it. Walk tall, swinging from the hips.

Making Progress

A long-standing disability may take longer to cure than one which has been a trouble for only a short while. As the pelvic floor becomes stronger, it will be able to resist increasing stresses.

Be content to make progress very gradually. There may be moments when some exertion catches you out without warning, and with insufficient time to prepare for it by bracing up. There is no reason to get depressed because you still find yourself damp occasionally. In fact, you may be coping far better than you did before starting to exercise regularly.

It is natural for women's pelvic floors to be slacker just before the menstrual period, owing to the cyclic effect of the hormones secreted by the ovaries. They tighten up again in the week afterwards, when more progress can be expected.

When at home prolong the intervals between bladder voidings. When you feel the first urge to empty do not rush towards the loo. Make your supportive muscles work more strongly to stop yourself going. Tell yourself firmly: 'It is not yet necessary. I can hold it a little longer'.

Acquiring any new habit takes time. Look on it as recreation—literally re-creation—and enjoy it!

After Two Months

Test your ability to restrain the bladder:

Stand upright with feet and legs *together.*

Brace up the pelvic floor and keep it braced.

Jump up and down on the spot three times—then stop and relax.

If you have leaked at all, continue with all the previous exercises, but leave this testing one out for another month; then try again.

When you can do it and remain dry, splendid! Go on with all the exercises for another month, then try:

The Final Progression

Stand upright with feet and legs *astride.*

Brace up the pelvic floor and hold it.

Jump up and down, with feet alternatively together . . . apart . . . together . . . apart . . . together . . . apart.

When you can do this with the bladder near to capacity and remain dry, put yourself to the final test:

On your guard—exertion is coming—hold the stopper tightly with the counter-brace—Now, cough hard! When you can do *that,* without a trace of moisture, you are cured.

Resolve never to let a day go by without consciously *using* your pelvic floor muscles in their supportive and stop-tap roles. You must maintain their strength, now that it has returned. Regular physical activity in a group is beneficial for most of us. But beware of strenuous movements which could strain both back and pelvic floor:—lying on the back and either raising *both* legs off the floor at the same time, or, raising the trunk to a setting position. They should only be attempted if you are *sure* that your pelvic, back and abdominal muscles are really strong. Even then, to be safe, the lower back should be pressed down and the pelvic floor braced up and held at the moment of lift-off.

Even elderly people can retrain themselves successfully, though it is likely to take them longer. One, a 73-year-old, reported having suffered from stress incontinence for fifteen years. By following through the described scheme of exercises, control and self-confidence were restored. 'Ah!', the reader may be thinking, 'But did it last?' Well, after four years the control is still being maintained—even on cold winter days!

It is never too late to improve muscles as long as it is possible to move them!

Protective Clothing

Nonporous material (e.g. rubber or plastic) should not be worn. Self-control is not increased through the knowledge that one is completely protected from embarrassment!

The skin reacts unfavourably to a greenhouse atmosphere. In the groin, there are numerous sweat glands, and if air cannot circulate around the skin, it becomes soggy and unhealthy. After a time, the nerve-endings become used to the feeling of moisture, which—more often than not—is only perspiration which cannot evaporate!

Keep yourself reasonably safe, but not so artificially fortified that you can afford to slacken your own muscular hold on the bladder outlet.

Have plenty of boilable cotton pants with a double gusset, fitting loosely in the crotch. If you go out for the day, take fresh ones with you, so that you can keep yourself as dry as possible.

If you are scared at the thought of a possible 'incident' on an important occasion, at a place where there will be no opportunity to change; then—and only then—resort to the impenetrable protection. Otherwise, don't even consider it.

While you feel vulnerable, get a little pocket made at each end of the gussets of your pants. Cut pieces of the gauze-covered absorbant rolls sold as liners for babies' napkins, and slot one of these inside. It will be there to imbibe, if necessary, while allowing the skin to 'breathe'.

Your control—like the babies'—will be less likely to improve if you come to *rely* on the padding; so, make up your mind to do without it whenever possible and hurry on the time when it can be discarded, completely,

Conditions having a Detrimental Effect on the Supports of the Bladder

Coughs

When lungs or bronchial tubes produce excessive mucus, the body endeavours to throw off the clogging deposits by forceful expectoration.

The abdominal and chest muscles contract to stabilize the rib cage, and the dome-shaped diaphragm, between the chest and abdominal cavities, moves up and down, in much the same way as a plumber's plunger when it is used to clear a stopped-up drain pipe. This action pushes the phlegm upwards, but it also produces a powerful thrust downwards.

The Treatment

If your breathing apparatus is obstructed, enlist your doctor's help without ado. But assist yourself with:
The Breathing Exercise. The emphasis is on breathing out. Imagine that you have to clean and polish a mirror without any agent except a cloth and your own breath. Begin by breathing out and making the noise you would make to fog up the mirror—but keep it up until all your breath seems to have gone and you can't make another sound.

Eventually, you will have to breathe in and the lungs will refill with air automatically. This movement will probably make you cough, so brace your pelvic floor in readiness and place your hands firmly on your lower tummy wall, to support it while you do so.

You may wonder why on earth—since you have been told that coughing is hazardous—should an exercise now be suggested which might make you do it? Well, the mucus in the lungs must be expectorated before your chest condition improves. The exercise helps the mucus to be cleared more easily and quickly, and the sooner this is achieved, the better!

Repeat this thorough breathing out—bracing your pelvic floor and tummy muscles as you force out the last gasp—four times every hour during the day, until your chest is in good condition. If you should wake up during the night, do it then.

Day-to-day Breathing

The activities of living are always performed better when the body-framework is well-balanced. Opposing groups of muscles which contract and relax to stabilize the trunk in movement, should always return it to a resting state of equilibrium, afterwards.

An attitude which imposes an unequal or prolonged strain on the muscular stays, will inevitably bring about unnecessary discomfort, fatigue and deterioration of function.

This applies as much to breathing—which for most of the time is unconscious—as to the consciously willed actions. Yet people with breathing difficulties are often to be seen standing or sitting in faulty positions:

1. The slouch—with forward-tilted pelvis, hollow lower back, protruding tummy and sunken chest.
2. The stiff-as-a-ramrod-shoulders-up-and-back type of carriage.

Both of them prevent full use of the lungs. Inspiration is restricted by muscular imbalance. Parts of the lungs are poorly ventilated, and with disuse, these areas become less healthy and more liable to infection (*Fig. 11*).

Correct use is what keeps our bodies in good condition. For a few moments, now, consider how posture influences your respiration. Think how you *are,* how your framework moves in breathing, and how you *can* breathe:

Get up and sit down again comfortably with thighs supported. Release the tension in your tummy and lower back. Place the backs of your hands against the *back* of your rib-cage, with fingertips almost touching. (Do not place the palms of the hands on your ribs, or you will arch your back and elevate the shoulders.)

Each time you breathe out, sigh gently, letting the shoulders go. Feel the slight release of tension as the breast bone and upper ribs drop.

When you breathe in, feel your lungs filling up with air from right down in the bases. Feel the rib-cage expanding *backwards* under your hands; then feel the lower ribs spreading out sideways,

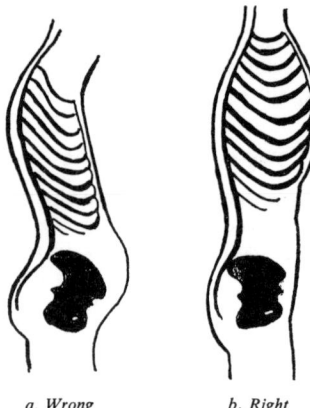

a. Wrong   *b. Right*

Fig. 11. a, Faulty mechanics. Trunk tends towards this form when its base (the pelvis) is tilted too far forward. It follows that: the back is excessively hollowed, the abdomen sags and the ribs droop—causing compression of the bladder (reduced capacity), the intestines (constipation) and inefficient ventilation of the lungs (susceptibility to chest infections and fatigue). b, Sound mechanics. Torso balanced, pelvis over hips (waist further back and perineum further forward than in (a). Chest cavity expanded without undue tension. Head and ribs eased up. Abdominal and pelvic organs have room to function well. Ventilation of the lungs is efficient.

then frontwards and upwards. Do it easily—smoothly—and relax again with a gentle sigh, as you breathe out.

If you will focus your thoughts on your posture and on breathing in this way for a short time each day, you will find, within a short time, that you are breathing more effectively—even when you are *not* concentrating on it!

Constipation

When the pelvic floor is beginning to respond to the retraining drill and tightening up, straining down at stools will retard progress. It might even undo the beneficial effects of the exercises already performed.

If affected this way, think about your diet. Are you eating enough roughage or fibre? One gets this promotor of easy evacuation from fresh fruit and green vegetables, wholemeal, wheaten, rye or granary bread, cereals containing their husks (bran) but not from refined cereals or white bread.

The Treatment

A simple natural treatment is to sprinkle whole bran on fruit or other cereals, though this does not suit everybody. If you still have trouble with hard motions—even when taking the roughage—ask your doctor for advice about laxatives.

Don't go for the harsh, purging medicines beloved by grandmothers! The effect is harmful. After taking them, the intestines require larger doses to induce another explosive bout of temporary activation.

The body should be allowed to keep to its natural rhythm—night and day—rest and activity—mealtimes and excretion of waste products from the bowel.

When the rhythm of excretion becomes upset—perhaps because on past occasions when the urge came, there was a train to catch or an appointment to keep elsewhere—a conscious effort should be made to establish it again. Give the intestines a chance when they want to move!

Posture is important, also, when emptying the bowels. Uncivilized people squat with thighs in contact with the abdominal walls on both sides. The pressure produced stimulates the wave-like movements of the intestines, which lead to easy evacuation.

Unfortunately, within the last century, the designers of modern sanitary equipment have made lavatory seats higher and higher. The result is that in our now-customary sitting position, that important stimulus is missing. It can be replaced simply and comfortably, in two ways:

At the usual time for evacuation, either:

1. Place a low stool, box or pile of old books in front of the lavatory (approximately six inches (15 cm.) high, but to be suited to individual leg measurements).

Sit down and place both feet flat on this support with knees apart.

Lean forwards until the thighs are in contact with the abdominal wall on both sides.

Relax, blow softly and maintain the position while waiting for it to happen. Don't hold the breath and strain.

Or:

2. When foot supports are not available. Place the toes flat on the floor, with heels up and knees apart. Clench the fists and place them in the groin on both sides, between the thighs and the abdominal wall.

Lean forwards and relax with the fists pressing into the tummy. Relax in that position and give it time to work.

Overweight

An excessive body content of fat is due to an imbalance between food intake and energy expenditure. The calories taken, over and above an individual's requirements are converted into fat and stored as fuel in depots underneath the skin. To lose weight, therefore, one must reverse the process and use up some of the hoarded fuel.

If one takes into consideration the necessity of eating sufficient nourishment for growth, tissue repair and the energy that has to be produced for the sort of life one lives, it is not just the amount of food eaten that counts. It is the type of food that matters, even more.

Certain carbohydrate foods containing refined sugars and starches have been proved to lead to an increased food intake, because they induce the feeling of hunger to return more quickly. Therefore the appetite is increased.

People who are prone to eating between meals—biscuits, cakes and sweets—often, without realizing it, become 'carboholics'. When these people change their diet and substitute with natural unrefined carbohydrates in the form of vegetables and fruits, their hunger is relieved for longer periods and they don't want to nibble between meals or to eat as much at proper mealtimes.

The Treatment

REGULATE YOUR EATING HABITS

Reduce your intake of refined sugars and starches, and you will consequently reduce weight and strain on the pelvic floor muscles, making it easier for them to function efficiently.

This does not mean going hungry! With your doctor's approval, you can eat as much as you like of the foods in the white group. These things contain the proteins, fats, vitamins and minerals which are essential for fitness and health, but hardly any carbohydrates:

lean meat, liver kidneys, sweetbreads, tongue, liver and continental or low fat sausage, meat paté	poultry, fish, eggs, cottage cheese, low-fat yoghurt, milk, oranges, grapefruit, apples tomatoes and grapes	green vegetables, salads, oil for dressing salads or grilling (not frying)

Avoid completely, foods in the black group (except on the rare occasions when, as a guest, your refusal might upset your host or hostess). These things contain very little that is of nutritional value and are high in calorie value—of which there are far too many! Avoid all fried foods. Take them grilled instead.

pastry and puddings, chocolates and confectionery, Yorkshire pudding and batters, custard, blancmange and thick sauces, dumplings, doughnuts and buns,	macaroni, spaghetti and all pastas, golden syrup and treacle, jam and marmalade, condensed milk and ice cream, tinned fruits in syrup, biscuits and cakes,	potato chips and crisps, rice, sago, semolina and tapioca, sweet drinks— long, short, alcoholic or non-alcoholic

If you are tempted to fall for any of the black foodstuffs, just say to yourself, 'Which do I really want more—that meringue (or whatever), or to be slimmer and feel fitter to relish other enjoyments in life?' Immediately, the fattening food will seem less attractive!

You certainly do not have to deprive yourself of all the things that you like. Most foods in the grey group (and some others which are not mentioned) contain enough calories to produce energy, and taken with the foods in the white group, provide sufficient proteins, fats, vitamins and minerals to make up a well-balanced, healthy diet. You can get plenty of variety by including nourishing things from the grey group in your menus—but take them more sparingly than you have been doing.

nuts,
fresh and deep frozen summer fruits—cherries, strawberries raspberries, red and black currants, apricots, peaches, pears and plums.
root vegetables, pulses and jacket potatoes,
dried peas and beans,
dried apricots and prunes,
soya flour,
wheat germ,
sprinklings of bran,
peanut butter,
yoghurt,
cheese, butter, margarine and cream,
evaporated milk,
soups—clear or with vegetables passed through a sieve or liquidizer, (without starchy thickening).
wheat or rye crispbread,
bread—the minimum, either wholemeal, wheaten, granary or rye

PEOPLE VARY AND THEIR NEEDS ARE NOT IDENTICAL. Those who are very energetic burn up more calories. However, most mature individuals eat far more than their bodies require and in doing so, simply overwork their digestive systems and give themselves more to carry!

CHECK YOUR WEIGHT REGULARLY JUST ONCE A WEEK, at the same time of day, on the same scale, in approximately the same weight of clothing (or without any). Let this be your guide.

AIM TO LOSE TWO POUNDS EVERY WEEK (not more) If you are not losing, eat less and less and less! For a few people, it might be necessary to avoid all grey foods as well as the black, and stick to the white ones, for a time—until the pounds show a positive sign of slipping away.

WHEN YOU REACH YOUR TARGET (the weight that you should be according to the chart on the scales at your local chemist) you can break out—if you really want to—on just one day a week, allowing yourself to take the prohibited food or drink.

CONTINUE TO CHECK YOUR WEIGHT, regularly, and if it begins to go up again, cut down once more.

Eating is one of the joys of living—but life can be enjoyed so much more if one is in good form.

It is a mistake to lose weight too quickly or to carry slimming too far. A certain amount of fatty tissue is necessary for 'packing' the internal organs and holding them in place.

Underweight people with stress incontinence might well improve the condition by gaining weight.

Contemplating Pelvic Surgery

Preparation

A respiratory type of anaesthetic is taken far better if the chest is clear and one is breathing easily. If another type is chosen when you go to the theatre, it will still be an advantage—particularly if you are a heavy smoker or have a tendency to cough or wheeze—to get your lungs cleared, beforehand.

Coughing makes any tender part of the body hurt or throb. The pelvic area will be tender after the operation. So, clear your lungs:

THE BREATHING EXERCISE

This is preventive. It reduces your chances of coughing, when you may feel rather sore, by removing excessive mucus deposits, prior to the operation.

Repeat the forced expirations, four times every hour, until you are all set for the theatre.

PELVIC FLOOR EXERCISES

Learn and practice the basic exercises for the pelvic floor muscles with purposeful attention. They, also, are learned more easily beforehand, when there is no interference with normal feelings. Then, having become familiar with them pre-operatively, one takes to them like a duck takes to water post-operatively, when they are so important.

Following the Operation

On coming round, there may be stale gases in the lungs. Get rid of them quickly.

START RIGHT AWAY:

The Breathing Exercise, exhaling very thoroughly, four times every hour, in the way already described under coughs on page 18. Doing this helps to remove stagnant mucus and assists the exchange of carbon dioxide for oxygen in the bloodstream—so vital to health and healing.

Keep it up until you are allowed to be active enough to breathe deeply, without this conscious effort.

NB Don't forget to support the tender area with hands firmly placed, low down on your tummy wall.

Pelvic Floor Contraction and Relaxation Muscle tone and full function are restored more quickly if the pelvic supportive muscles are exercised—gently—as soon as possible. At first it may hurt a bit, but movements in the area—however slight—help to disperse the inflammatory products which collect, causing congestion, numbness and discomfort. A fresh supply of oxygenated blood is brought into the locality each time the pelvic floor muscles are squeezed and relaxed. In effect, it is rather like cleansing a soapy sponge in the bath water.

After a few contractions, the pressure on nerve endings is reduced, and one finds that the whole area feels more comfortable.

Repeat the squeezing and relaxing for brief periods, frequently.

NB If you do *not* contract those muscles at all, they are liable to lose tone and become weaker within two days!

Gosling* has shown that within the voluntary muscles of the pelvic floor there are two distinct types of fibre. One type is responsible for closing the passages forcefully and for resisting sudden rises in pressure within the abdominal cavity. They are able to contract quickly, but they also tire quickly. The other type is responsible for drawing up and supporting the internal organs. They are slow to contract but are able to remain braced for long periods without fatigue. It seems that if the particular function of

---

* Gosling, J. A. et al. *British Journal of Urology* (1981; 53;**41**).

either type is impaired, for example through surgery, each is capable of adapting (with practice) to serve the purpose of the other.

Temporary Loss of Bladder Control

This sometimes occurs after an operation and may be a nuisance. There are two types which may last for a short time both caused by localized numbness of the nerves:

1. INABILITY TO PASS URINE

For this, follow simple pelvic floor exercises with stimulation of the surface parts by warm water from a bidet or a shower spray, held in the hand.

Then try the old trick of suggestion—turn a nearby tap on and let the water run as you get ready to initiate the outflow.

2. INCONTINENCE

For this, after the exercises, cooling by means of ice cubes moved gently over the perineum can prove helpful (held in plastic film—not in contact with the skin or it may stick), as can warmth from an infra-red lamp or a covered hot-water bottle and warm salt baths.

In some instances, further medical treatment may be necessary, but pelvic floor exercises are especially important, right through the period of healing and in the convalescent weeks ahead.

On the Second Day

The following exercises should be added:

ABDOMINAL RETRACTION

You can do this in any position, whether in bed or up and out; lying, sitting, kneeling or standing. Pull your tummy wall inwards and backwards towards your spine, making yourself as thin as you possibly can, from front to back. Hold for a second or two—and relax.

Repeat once at a time, but OFTEN during each day.

After One Week

Further exercises should be added:
The four tail-wagging movements described on pp. 12–14, once daily.

Check and readjust your posture, from time to time during the day (*see* pp. 14–15).

Keep up all these exercises for six weeks, to ensure a complete recovery.

Even after that, make it a habit to *use* your pelvic floor muscles regularly, to maintain them in efficient working order.

Controlling the Frequency of Urges to Pass Urine

Through anxiety to avoid the risk of accidental leakage, a bladder may be voided more than necessary and consequently—if it is never *allowed* to fill—it shrinks. In that case, in addition to having the cause of its unruly behaviour investigated and, possibly, treated, corrective re-training should be applied not only to the muscular shut-off grip of the urethra, but also to the bladder itself. It can be made more capacious and less demanding, quite simply by gradually lengthening the intervals between emissions:

1. When the desire to void first makes itself felt, it must be resisted *very strongly* with the muscles of the pelvic floor. The effect of this is to make the urge subside quickly (usually within a minute) and it then becomes easy to postpone the release of urine. When this procedure is repeated regularly, the bladder slowly responds.

2. The times at which voiding actually occurs should be recorded by oneself with ticks on squared paper, using each square on a horizontal line to represent an hour and those on vertical lines to represent subsequent days. The effect of this is to encourage a competitive spirit and to build up confidence by *showing* improvement.